Healing Garden

Butterflies And Flower Gardens

Stress Relief and Relaxation To Promote Healing

charlotte berry

BIC Subject category: 1. Drawing-coloring books for grown-ups 2. Arts & Photography- techniques
3. Craft, hobbies- art 4. Self-help-art therapy & relaxation 5. Self-help-anger management. 6.Self-help-stress relief

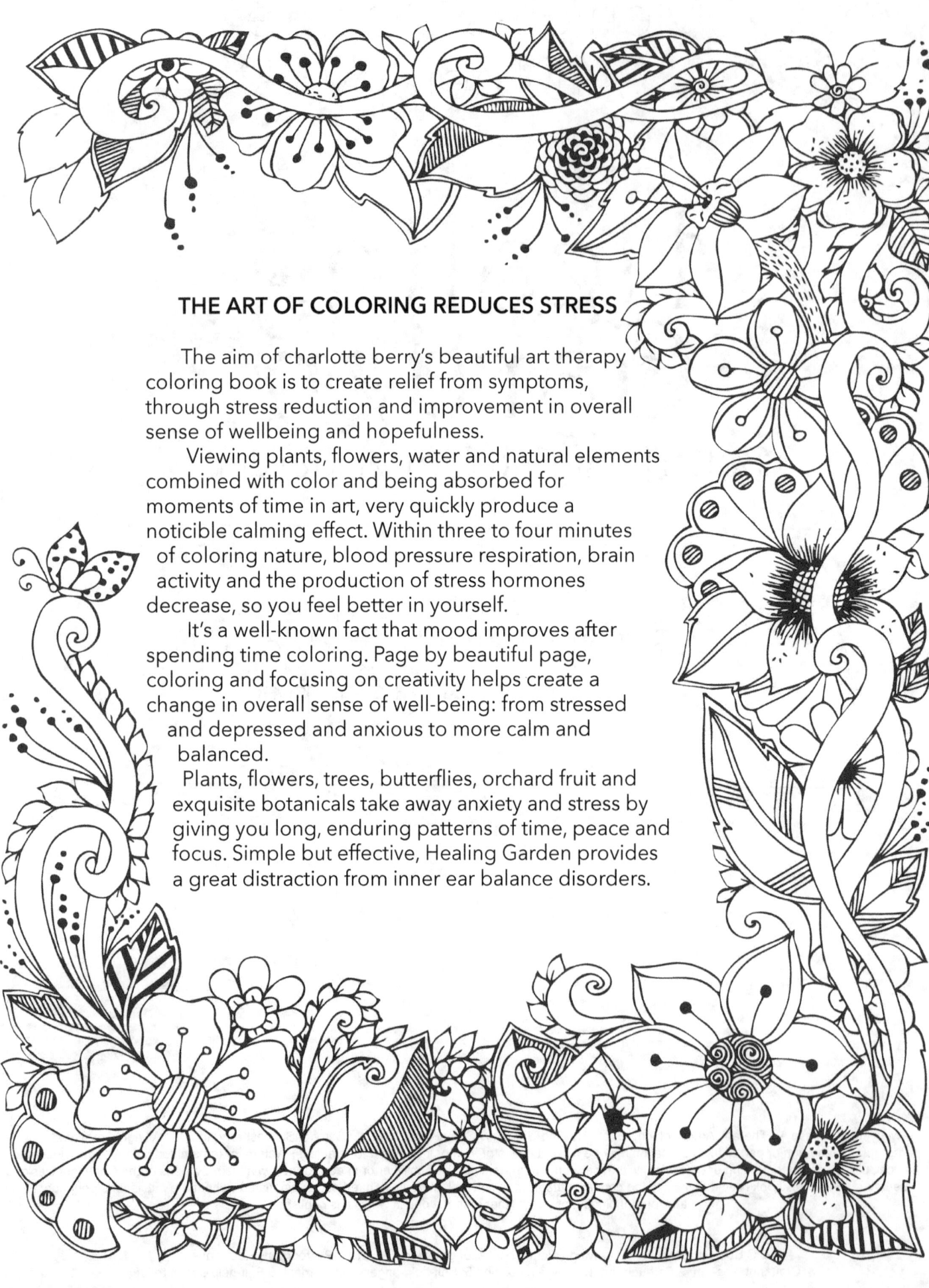

THE ART OF COLORING REDUCES STRESS

The aim of charlotte berry's beautiful art therapy coloring book is to create relief from symptoms, through stress reduction and improvement in overall sense of wellbeing and hopefulness.

Viewing plants, flowers, water and natural elements combined with color and being absorbed for moments of time in art, very quickly produce a noticible calming effect. Within three to four minutes of coloring nature, blood pressure respiration, brain activity and the production of stress hormones decrease, so you feel better in yourself.

It's a well-known fact that mood improves after spending time coloring. Page by beautiful page, coloring and focusing on creativity helps create a change in overall sense of well-being: from stressed and depressed and anxious to more calm and balanced.

Plants, flowers, trees, butterflies, orchard fruit and exquisite botanicals take away anxiety and stress by giving you long, enduring patterns of time, peace and focus. Simple but effective, Healing Garden provides a great distraction from inner ear balance disorders.

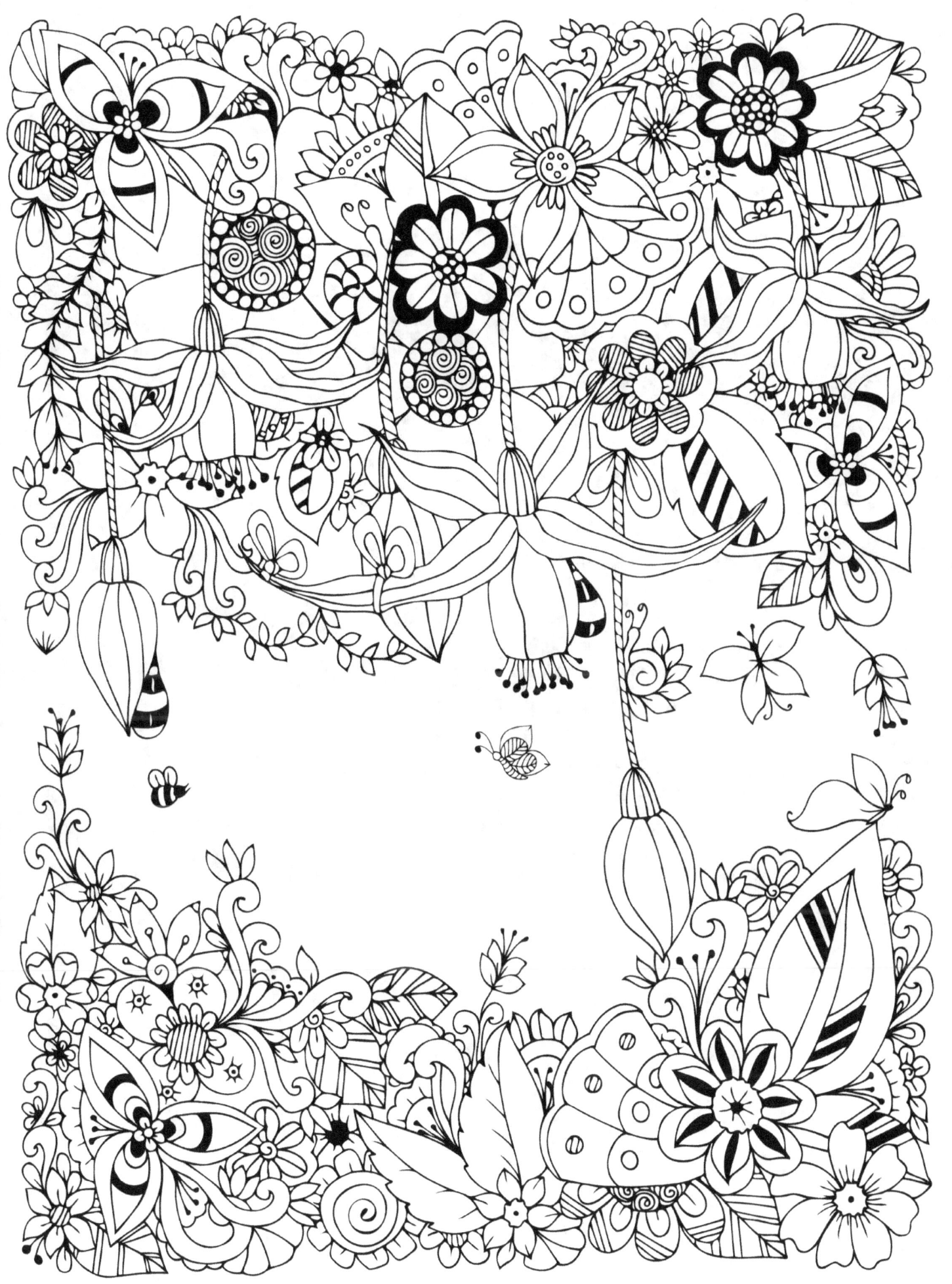

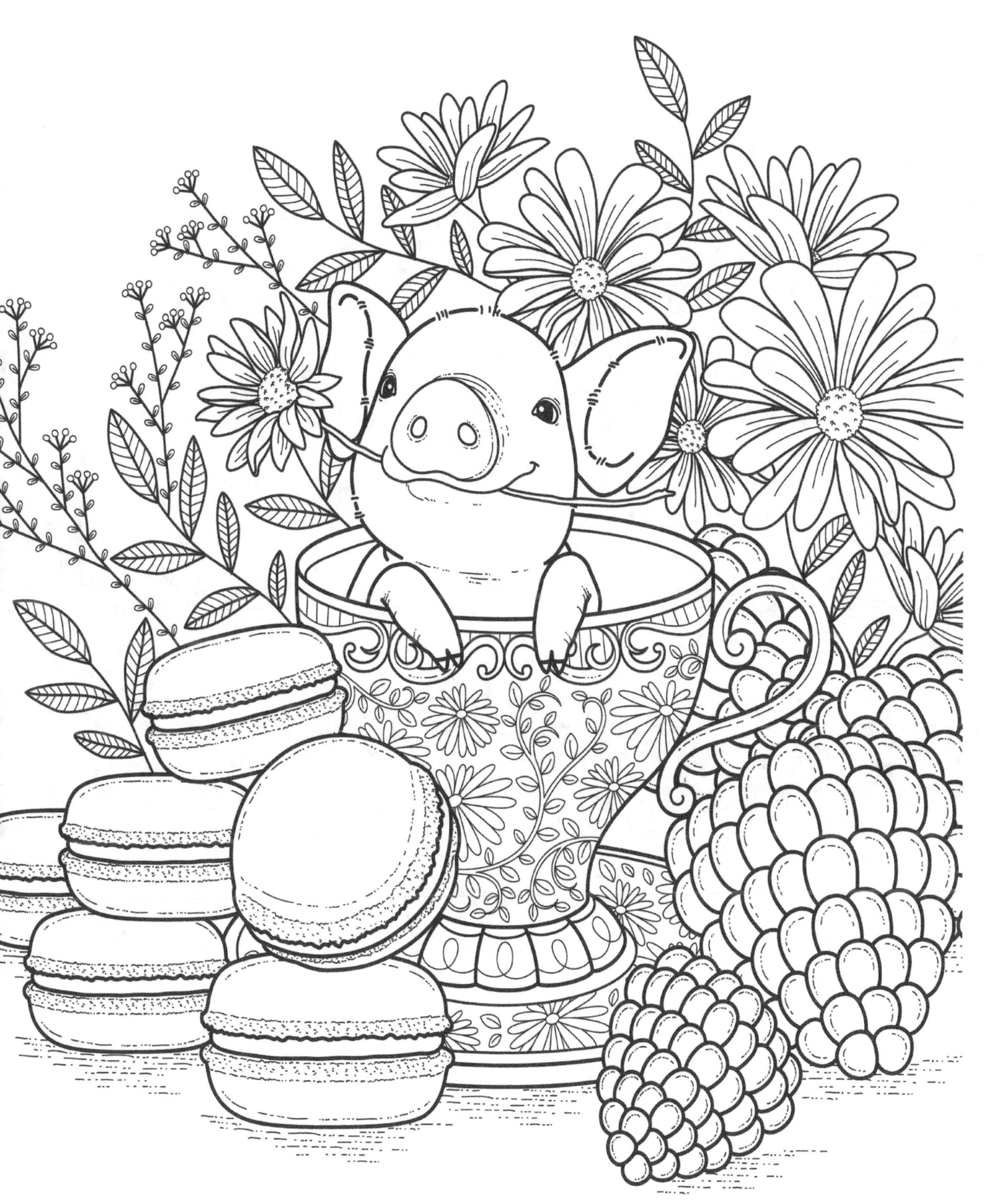

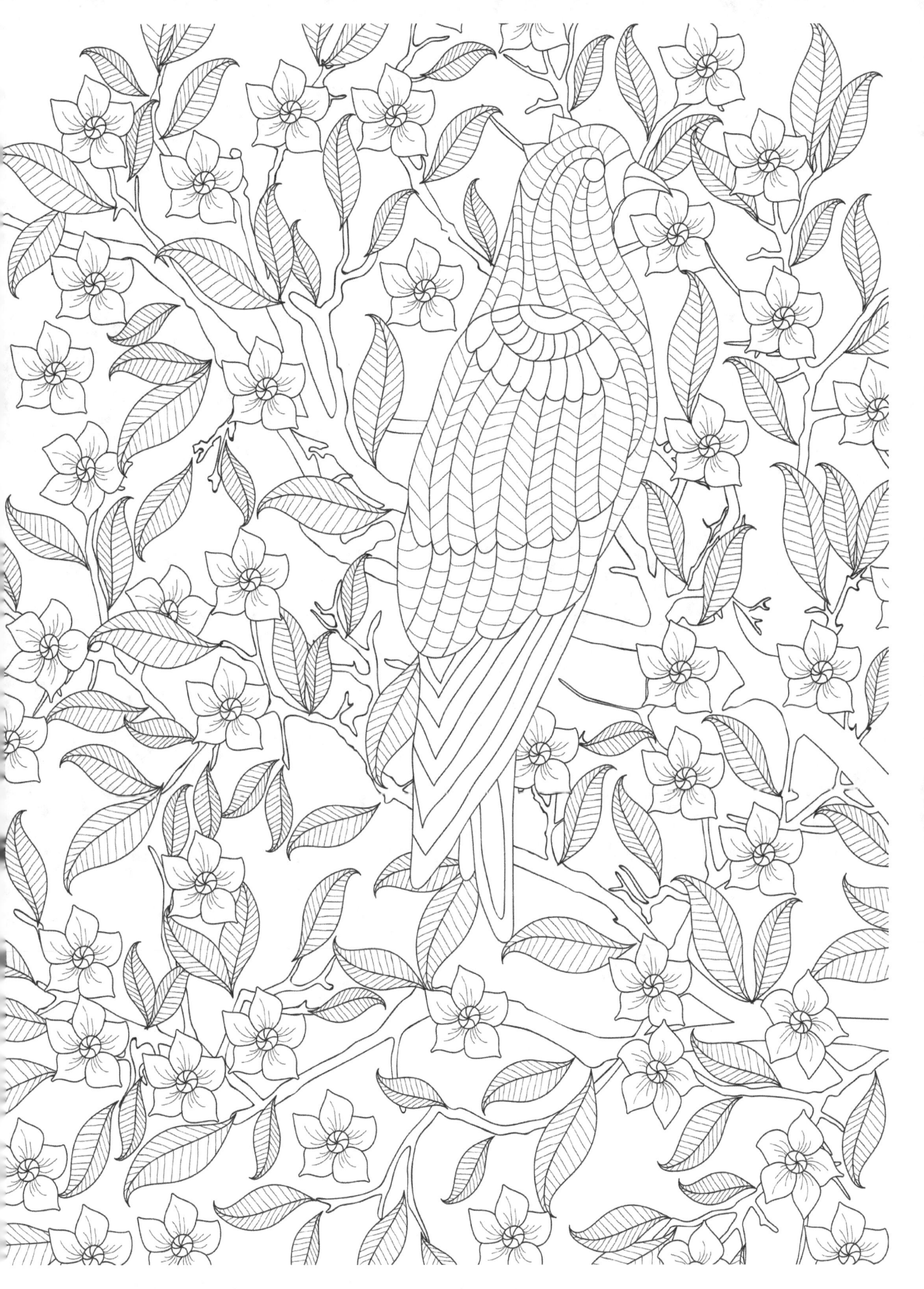

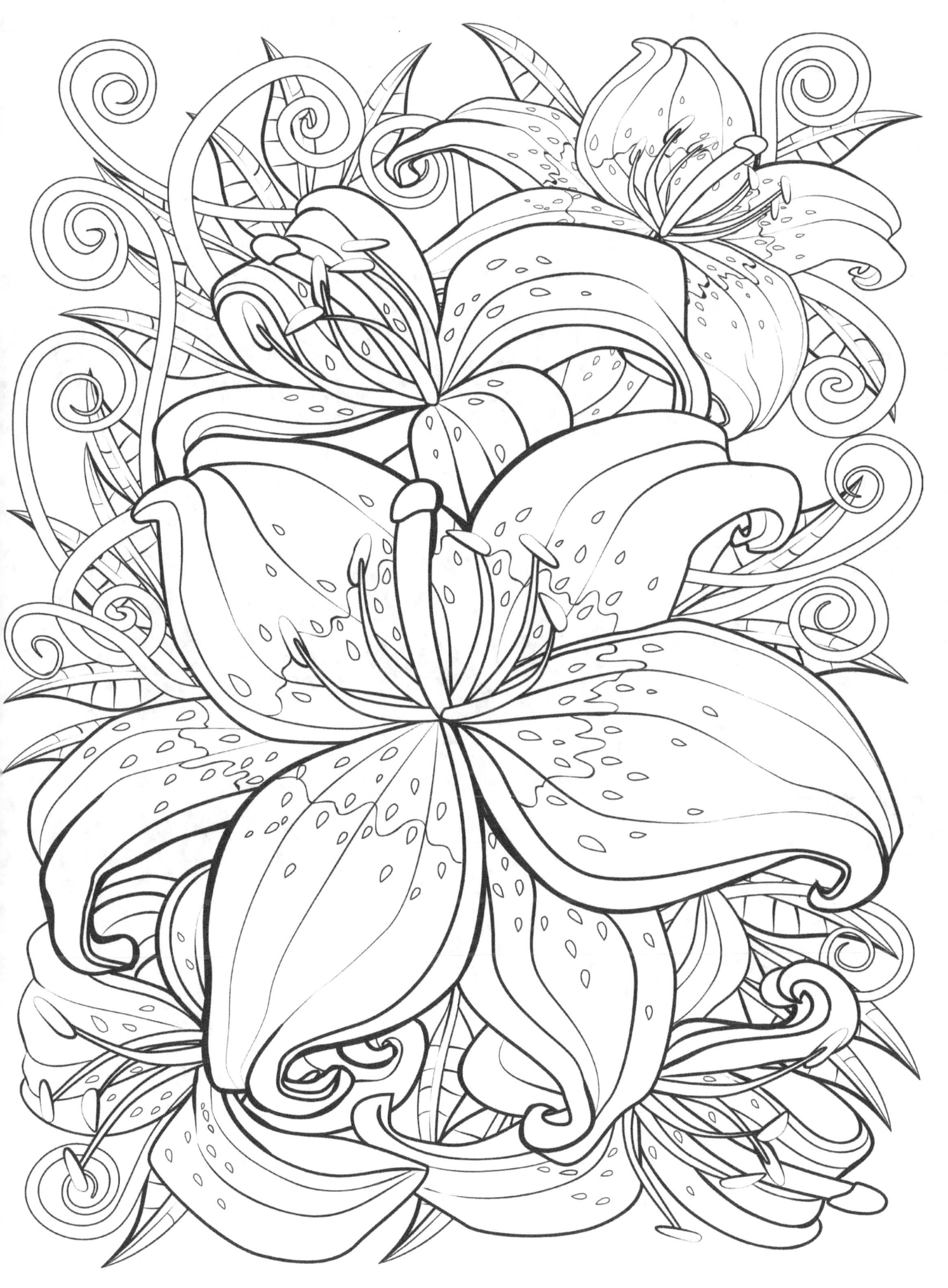

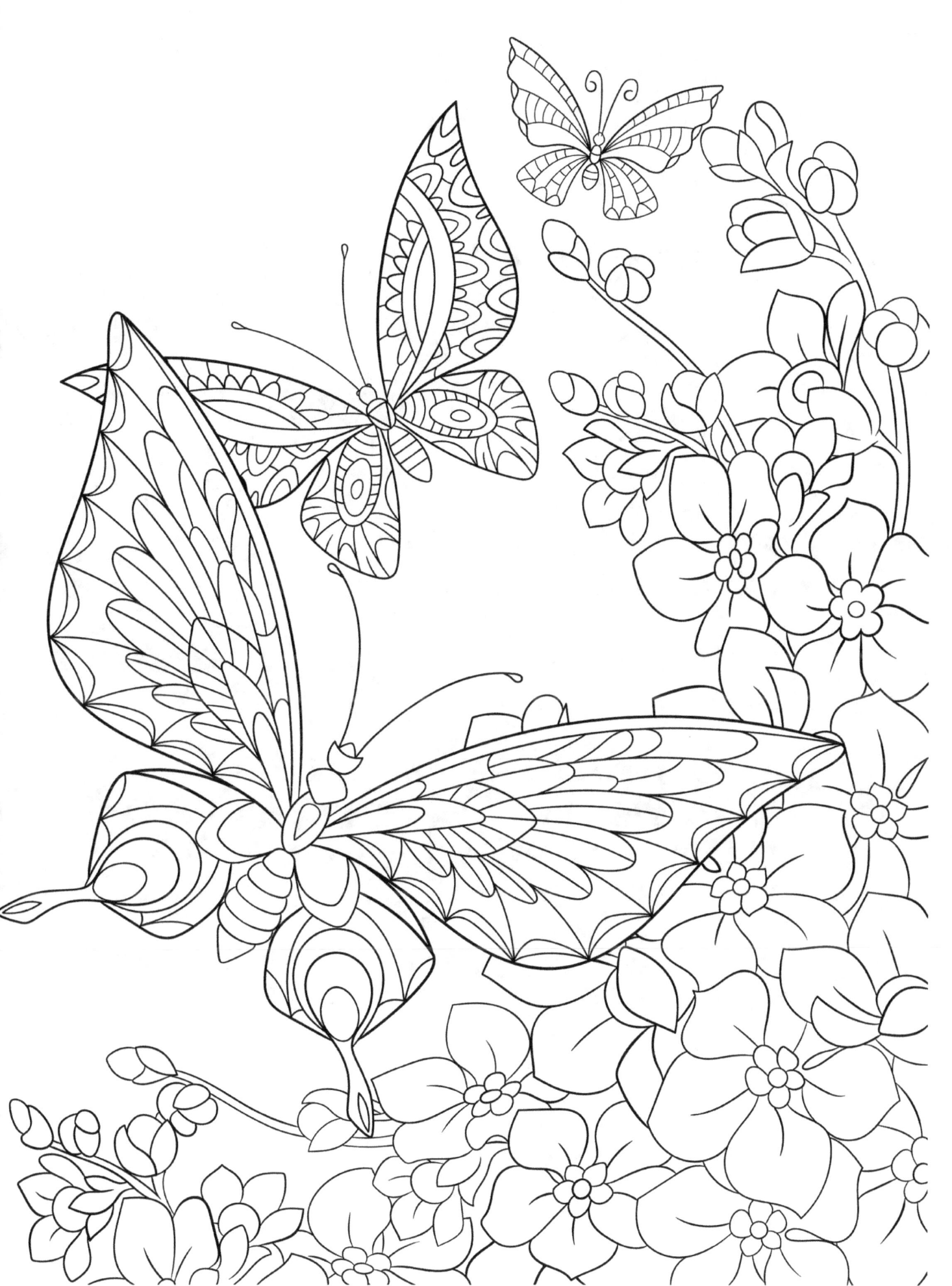

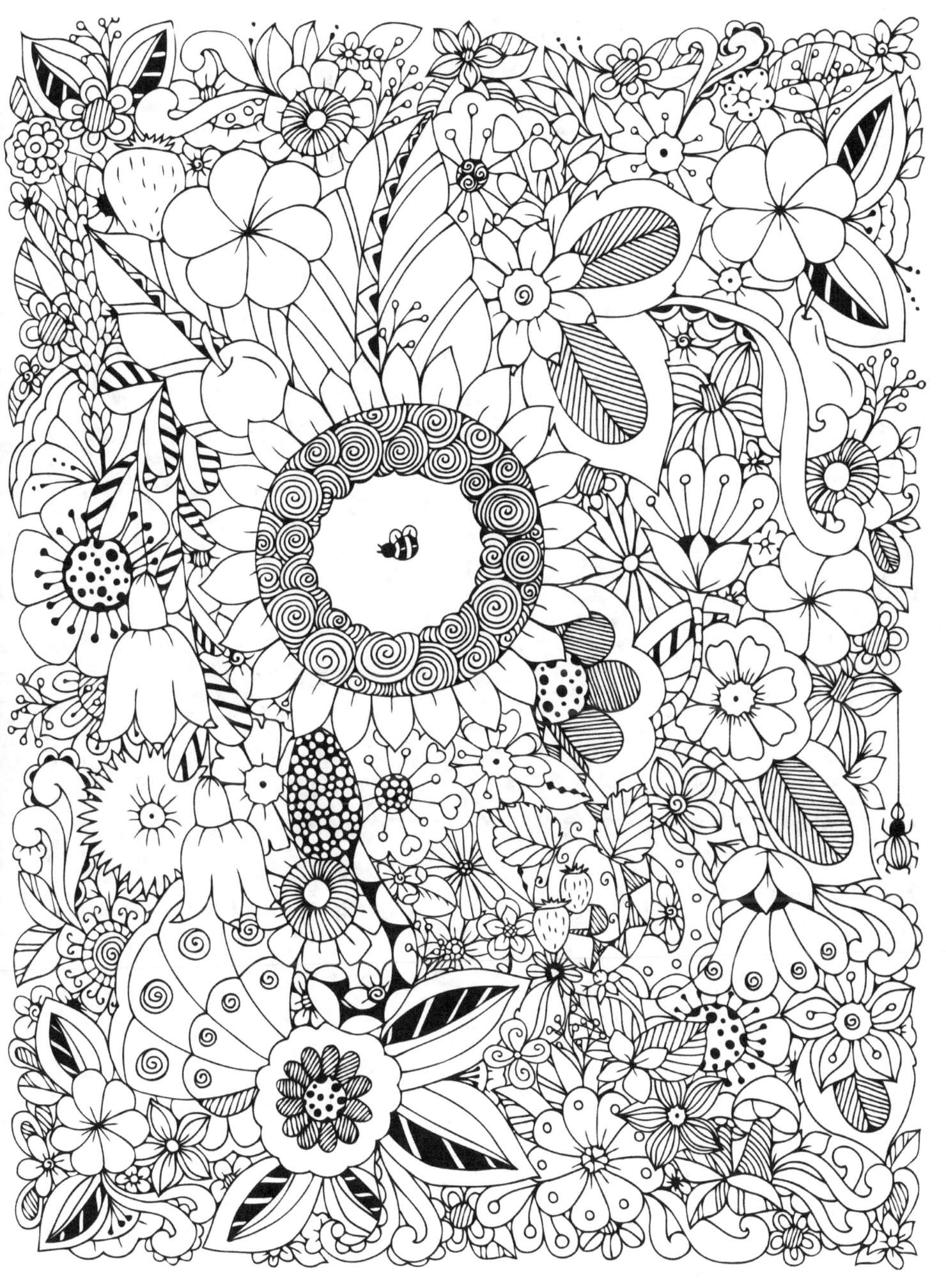

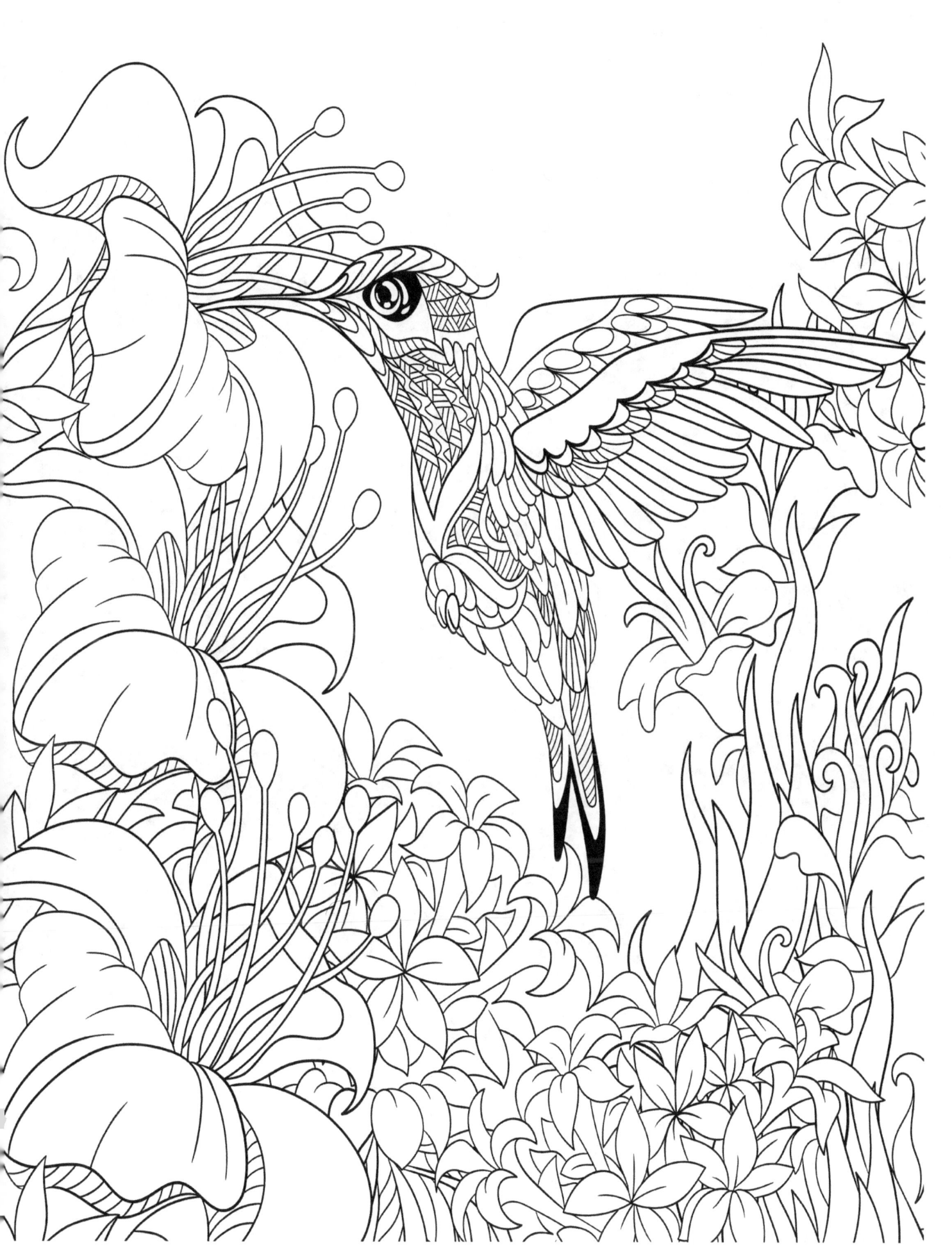

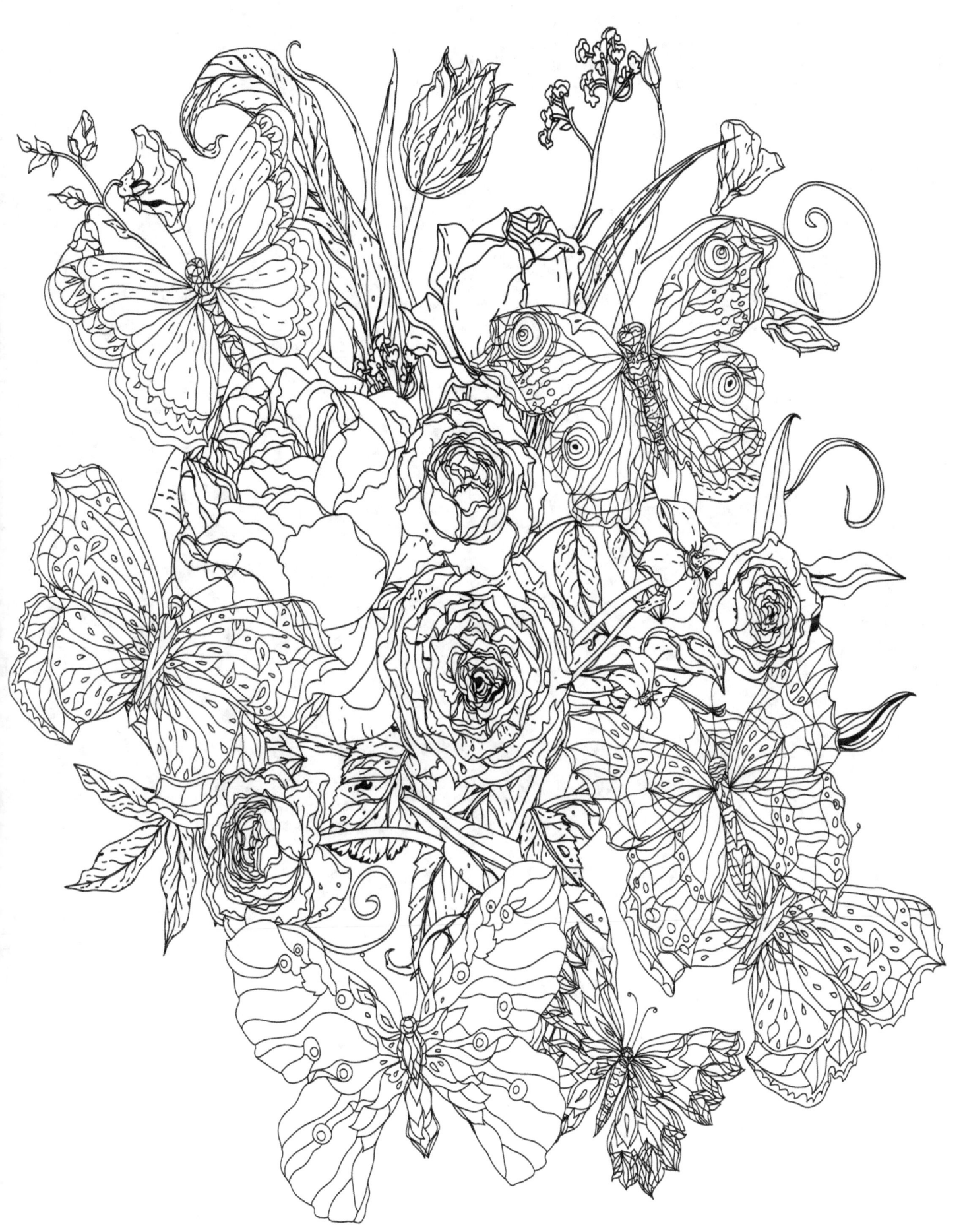

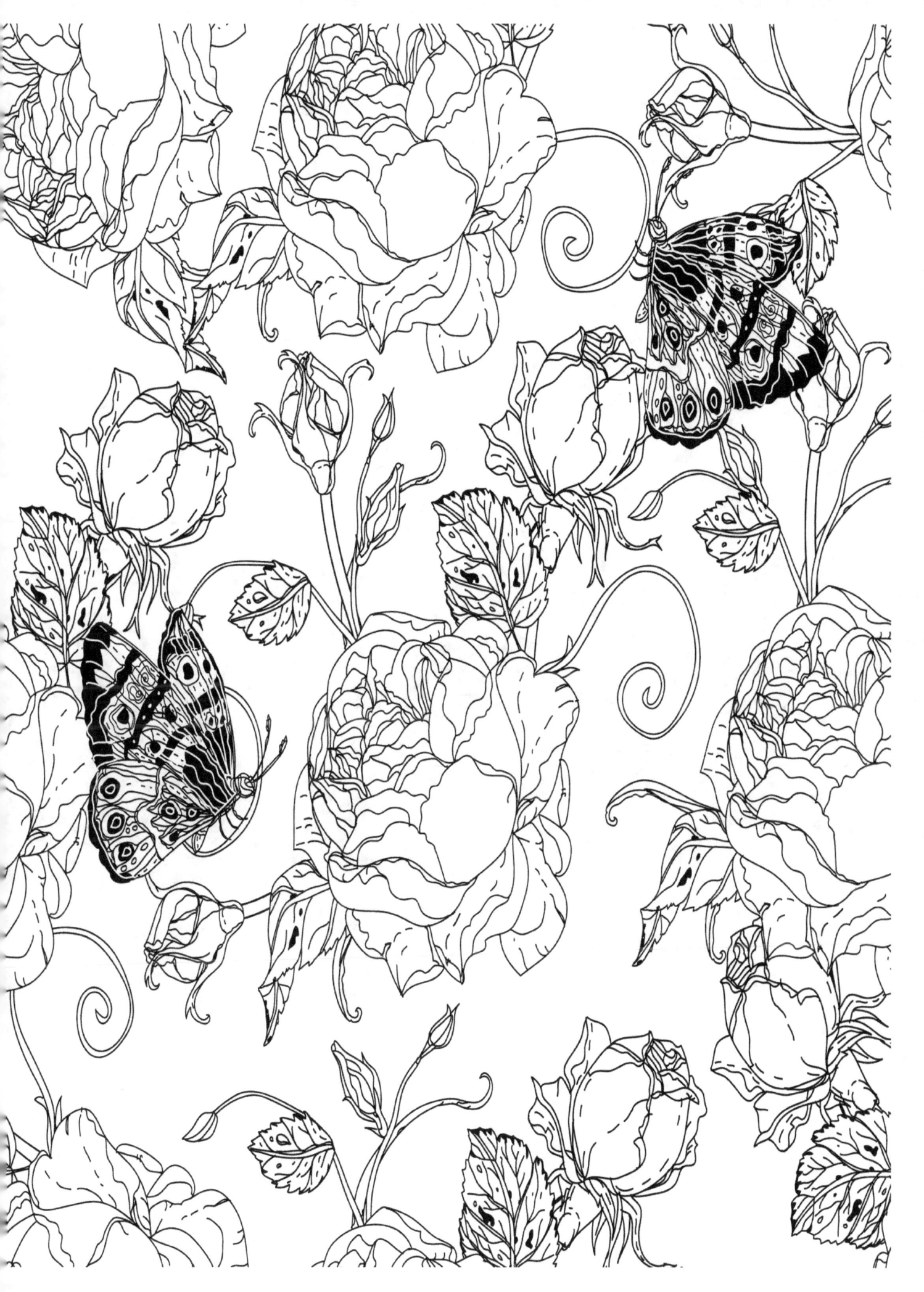

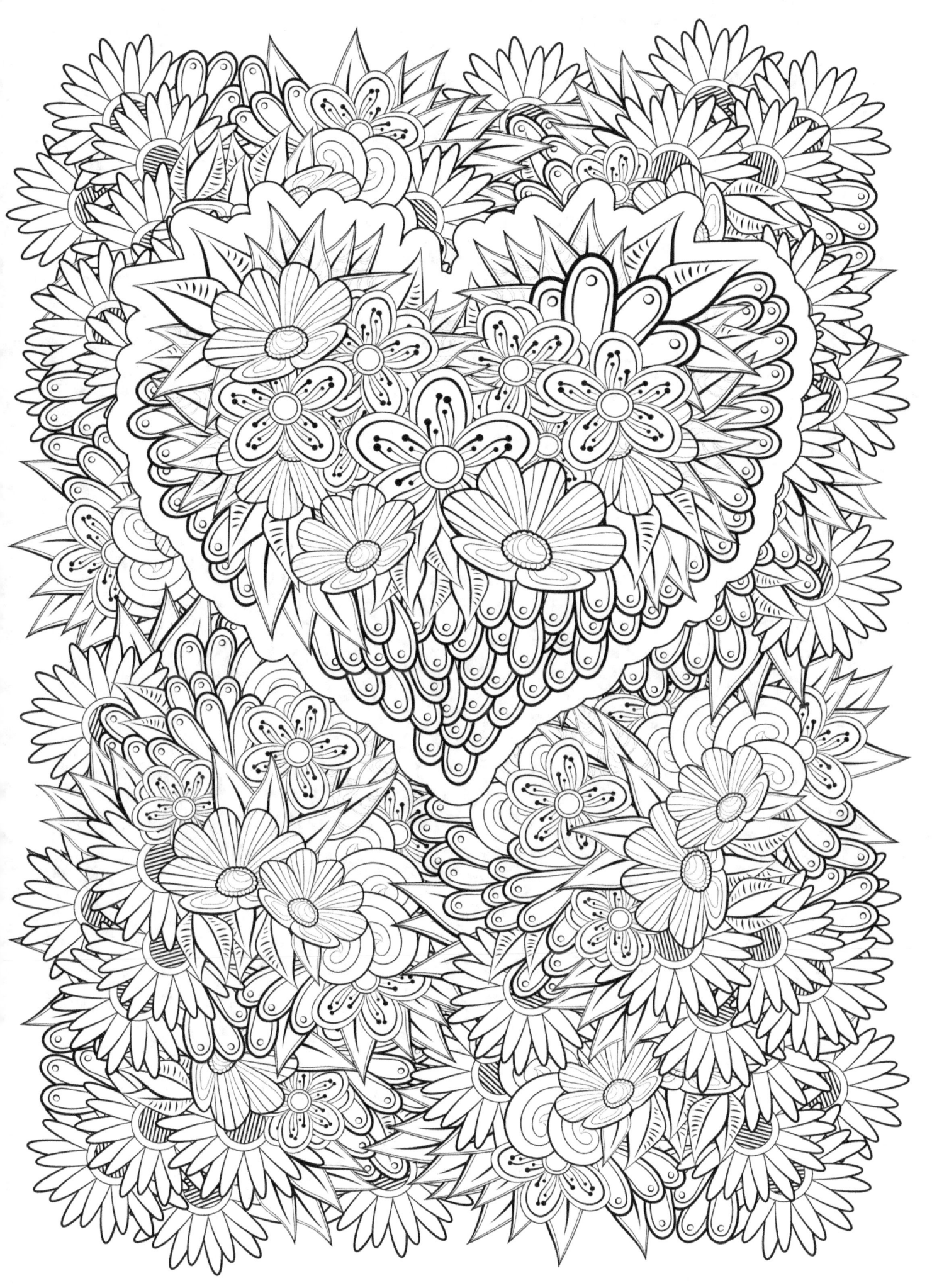

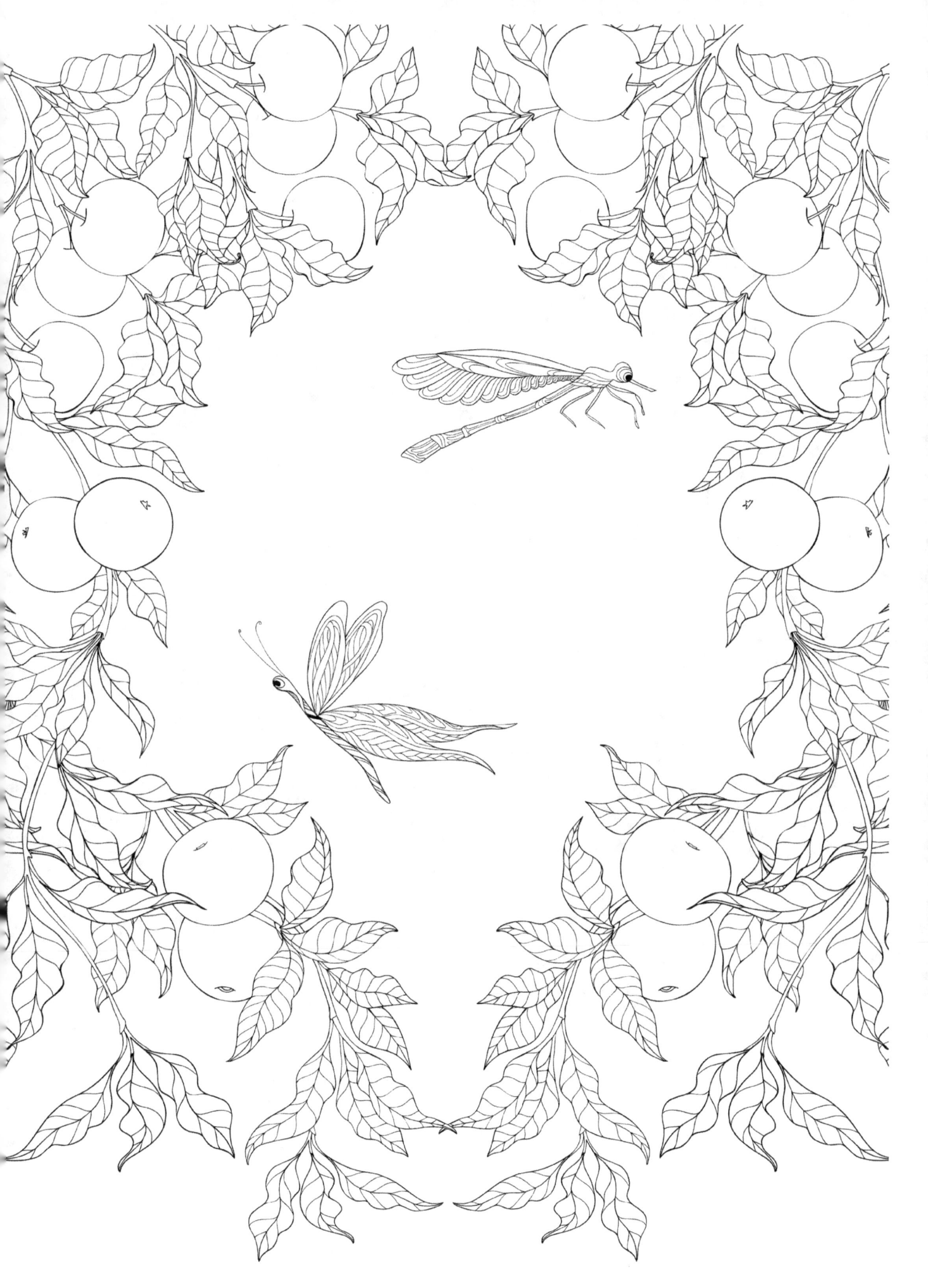

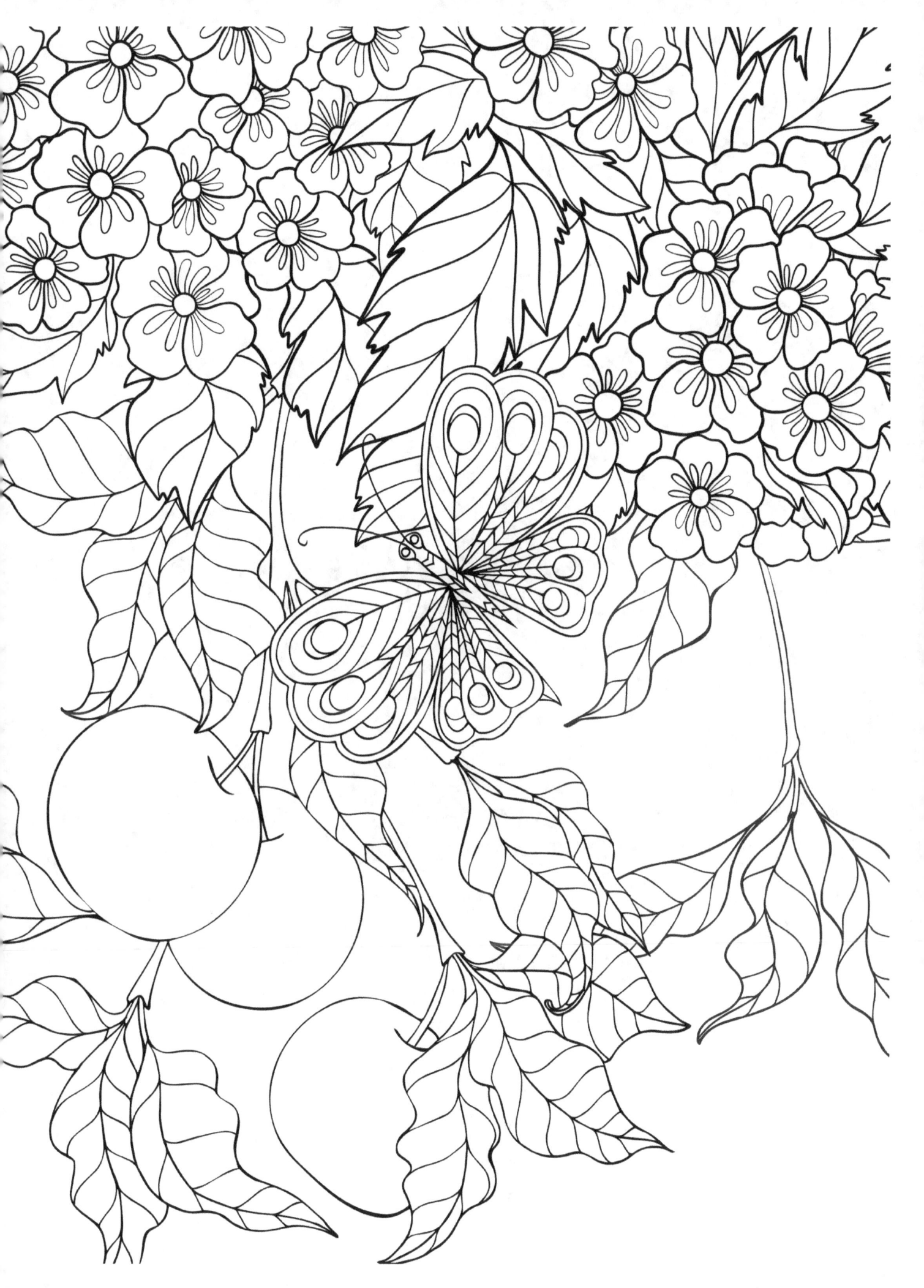

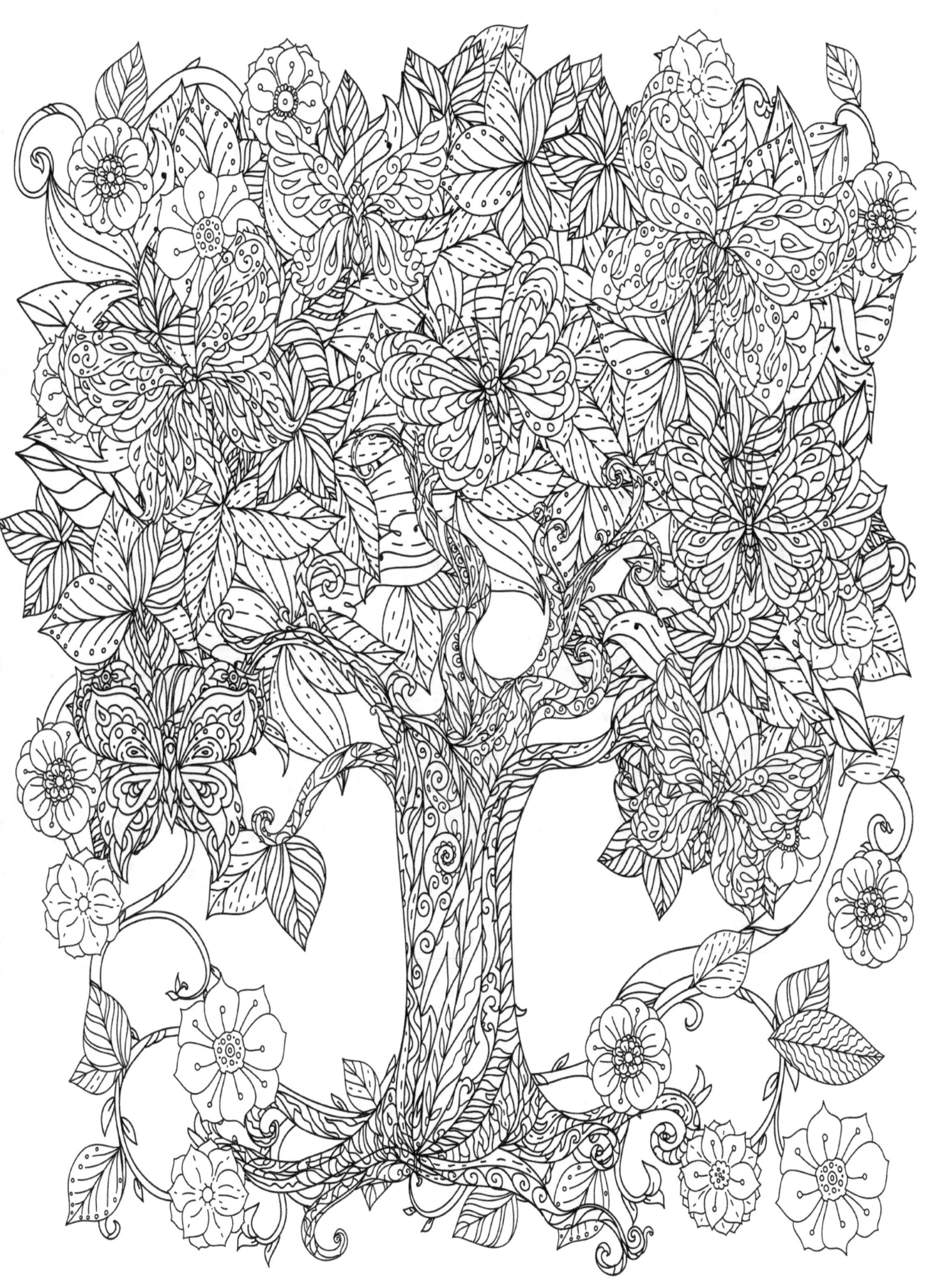

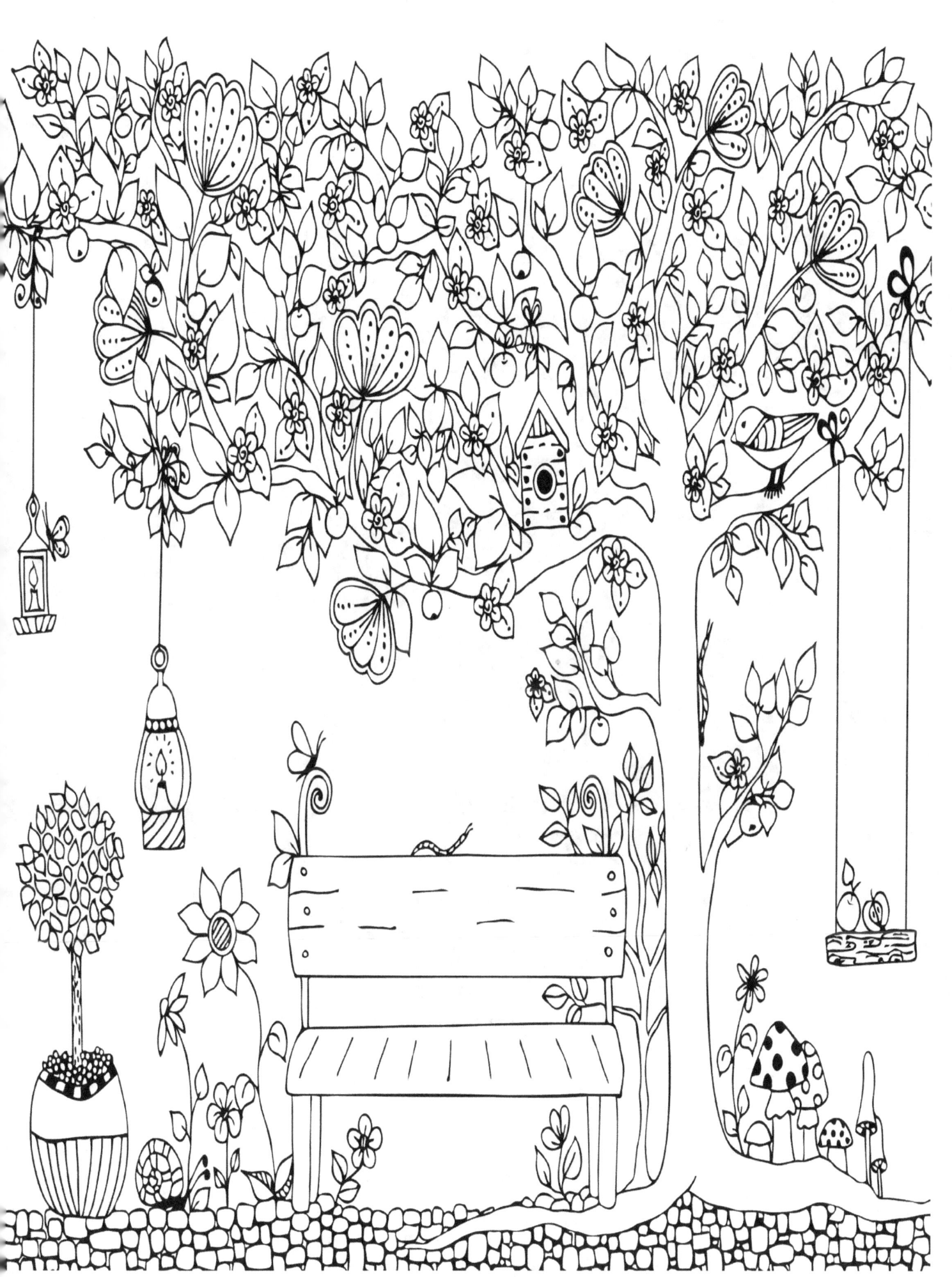

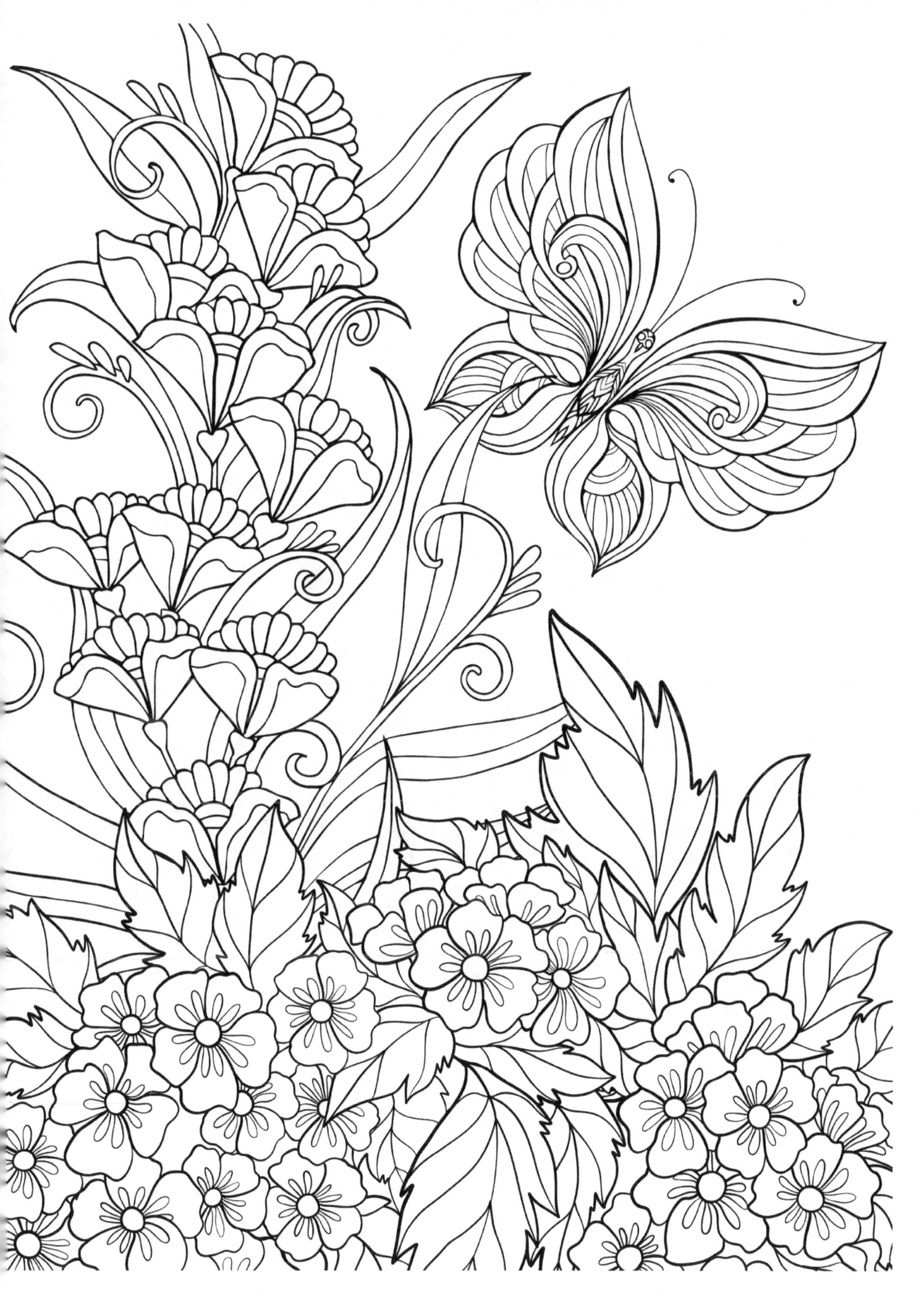

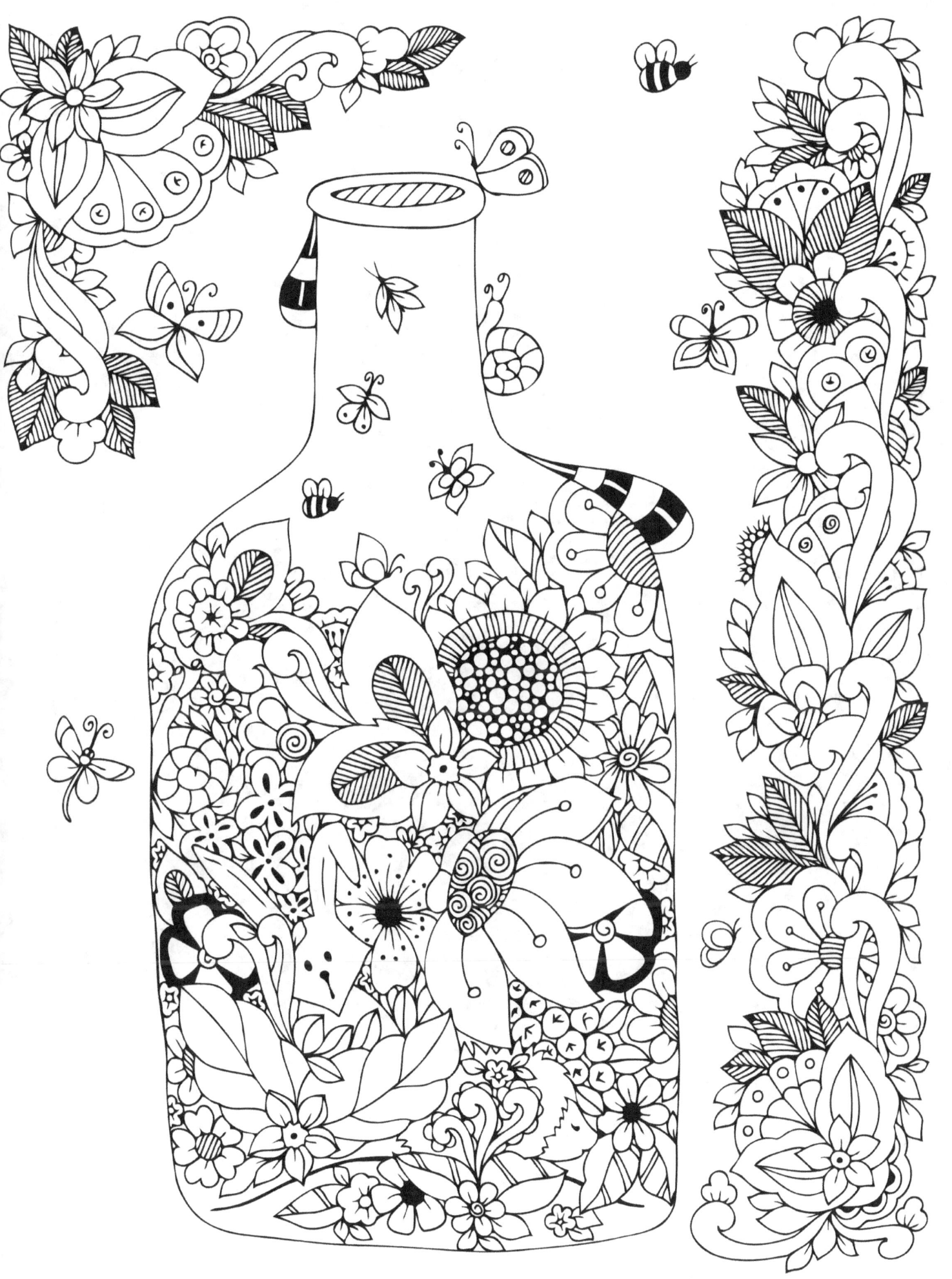

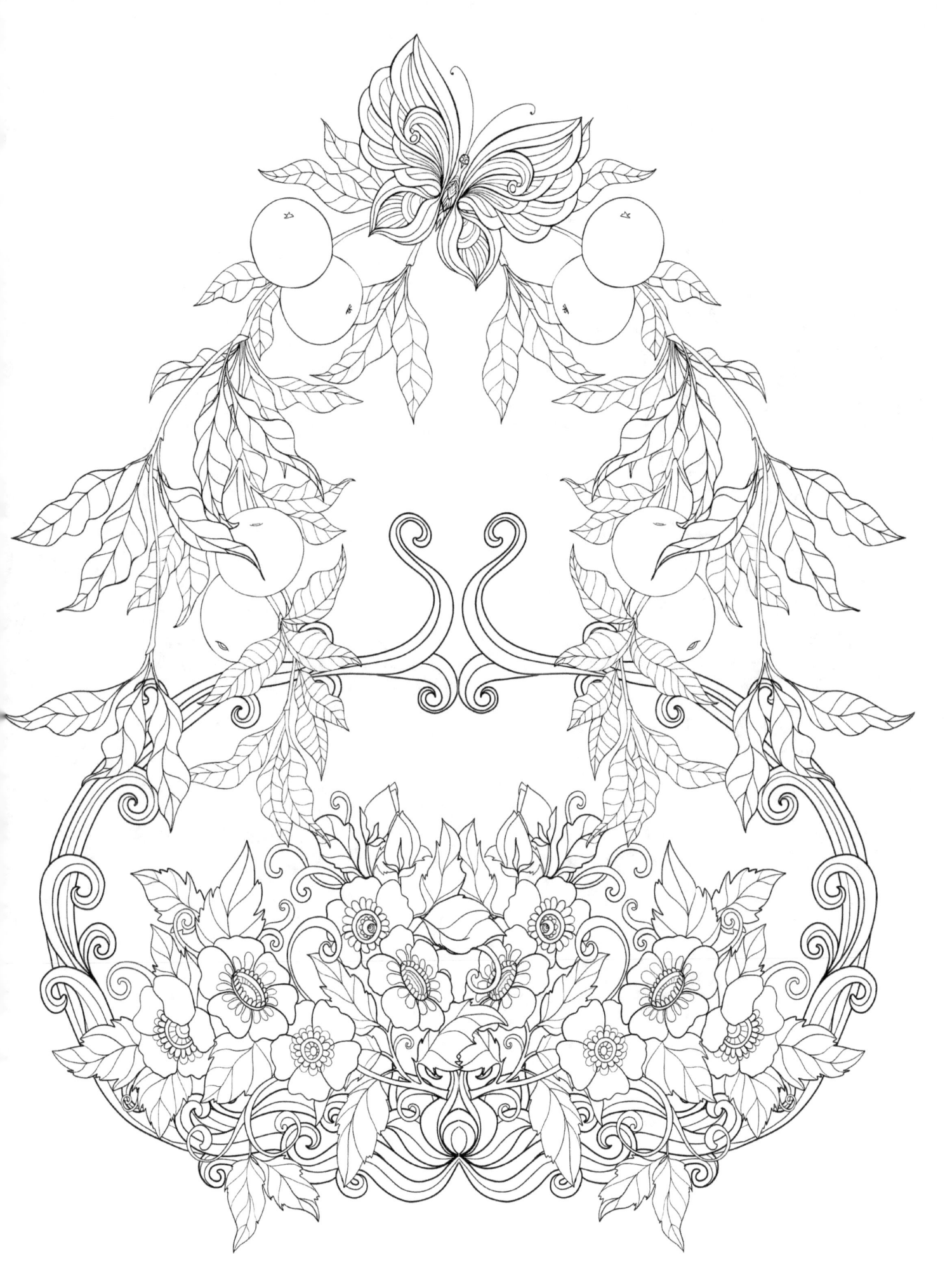

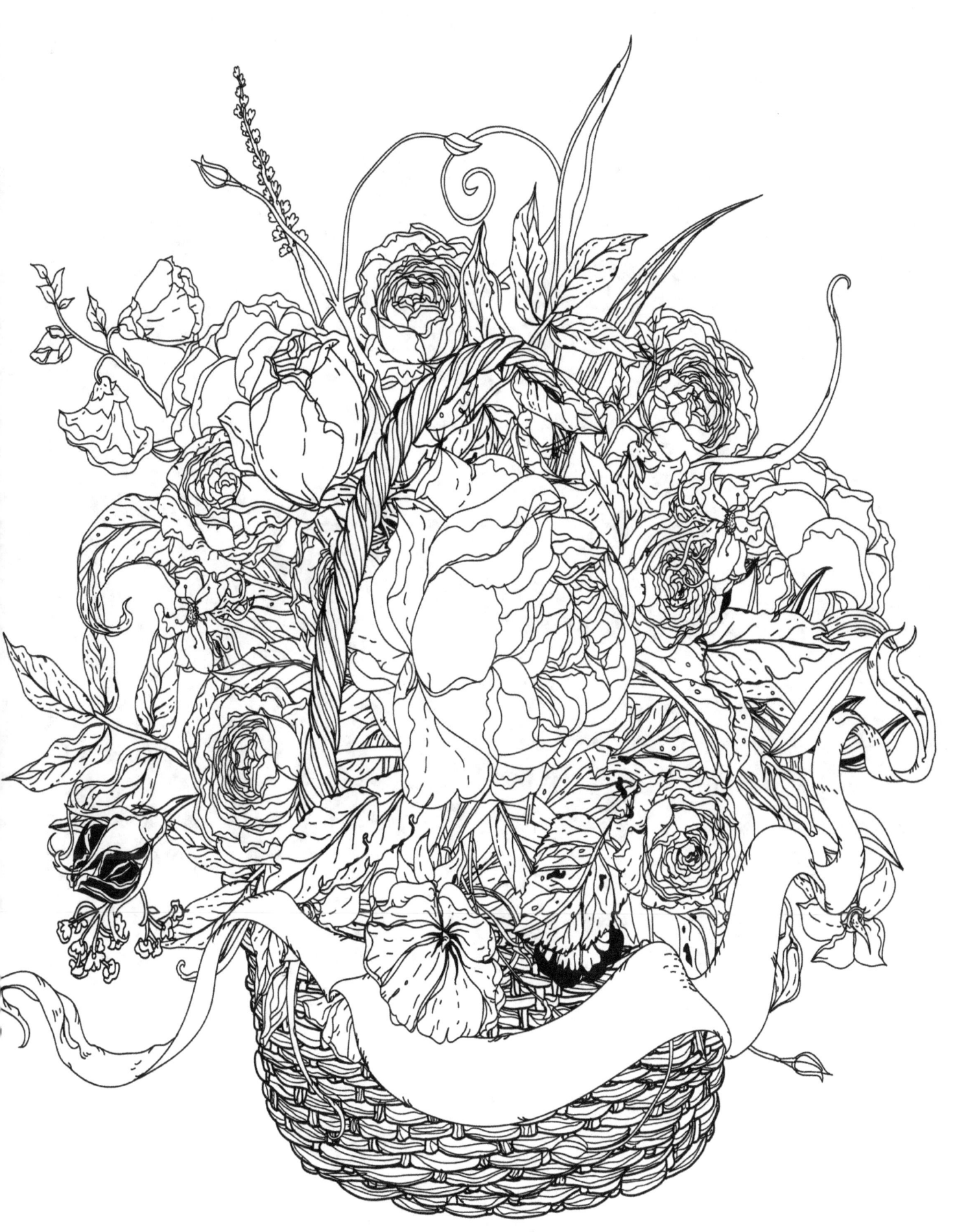

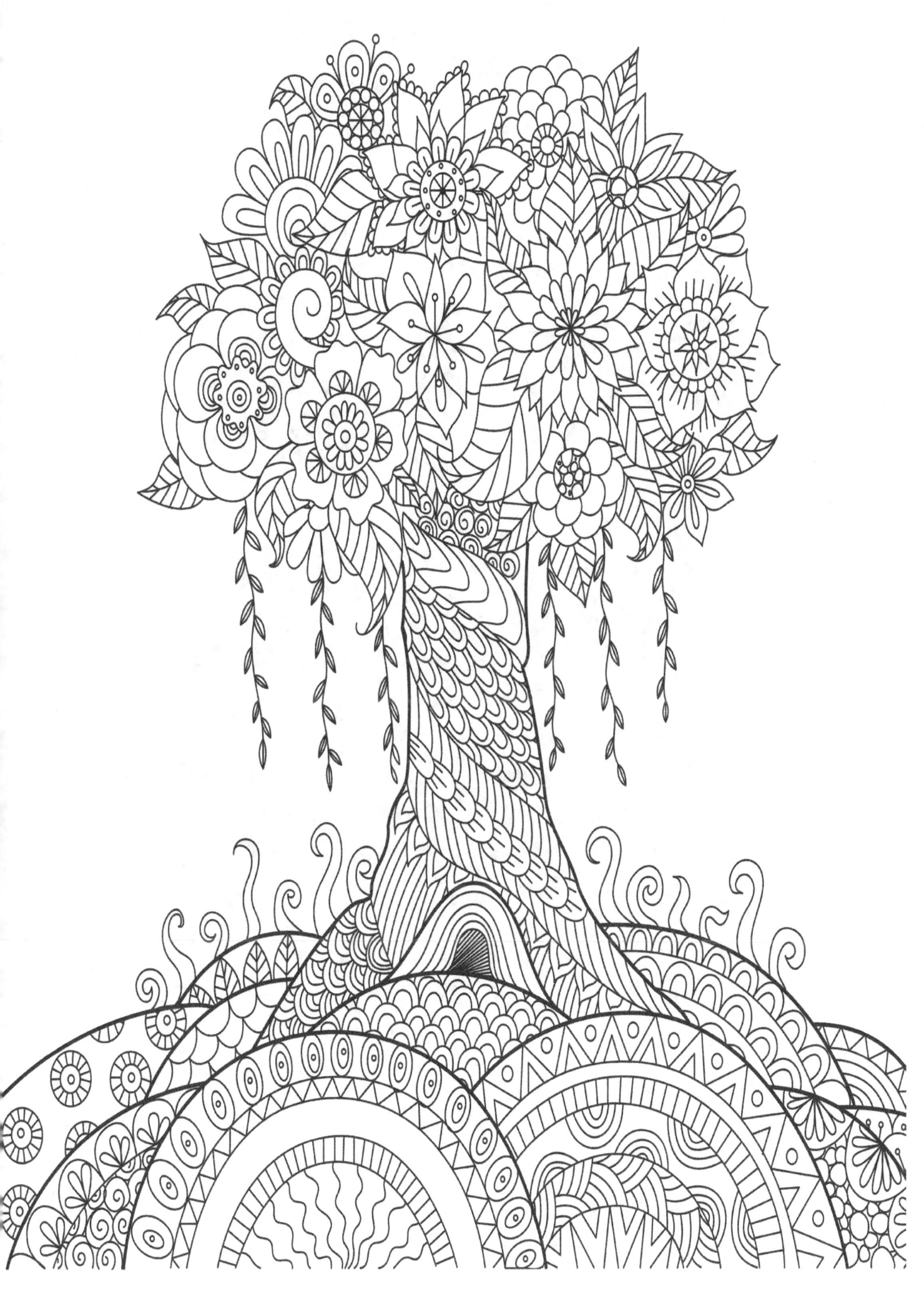

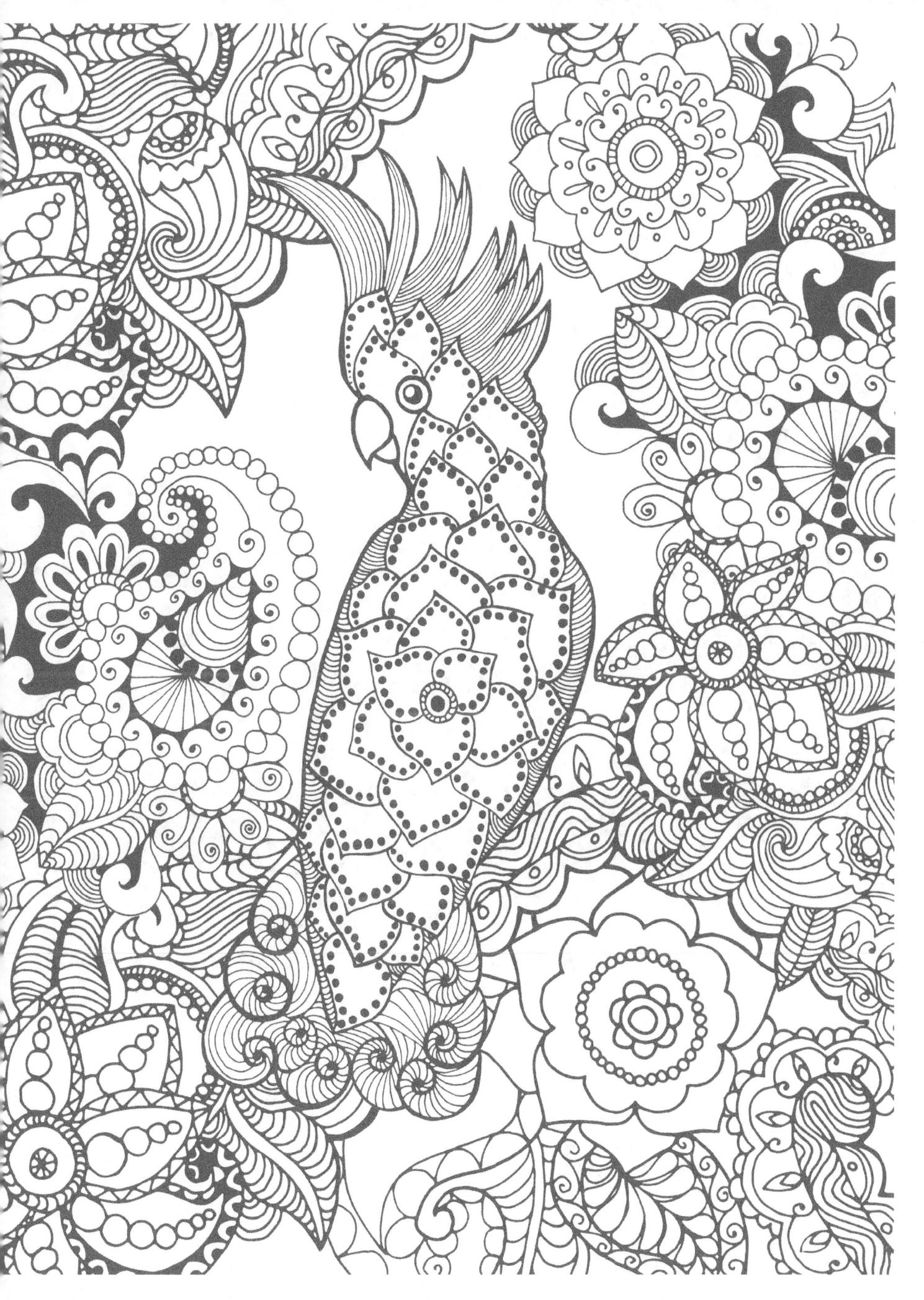

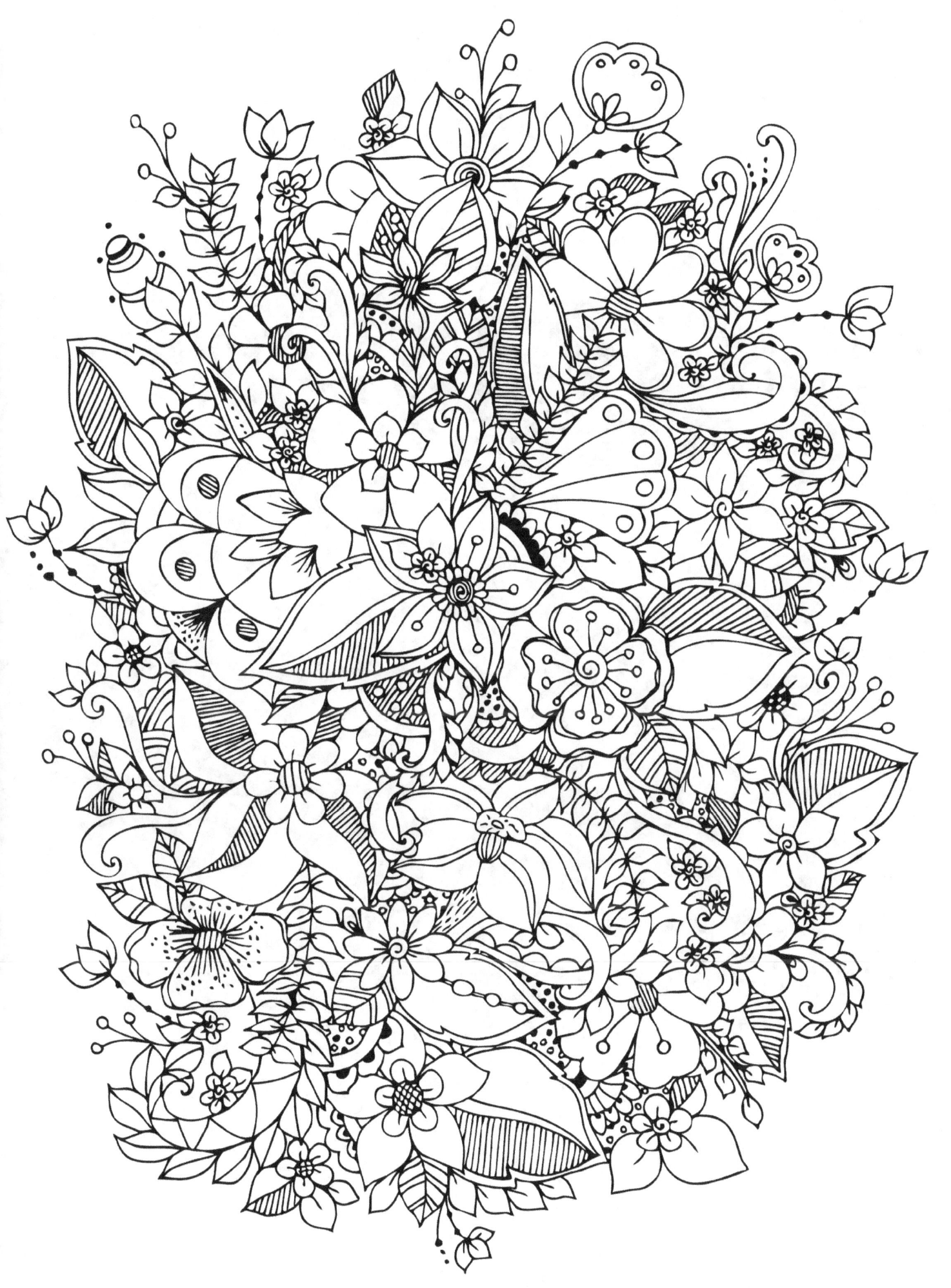

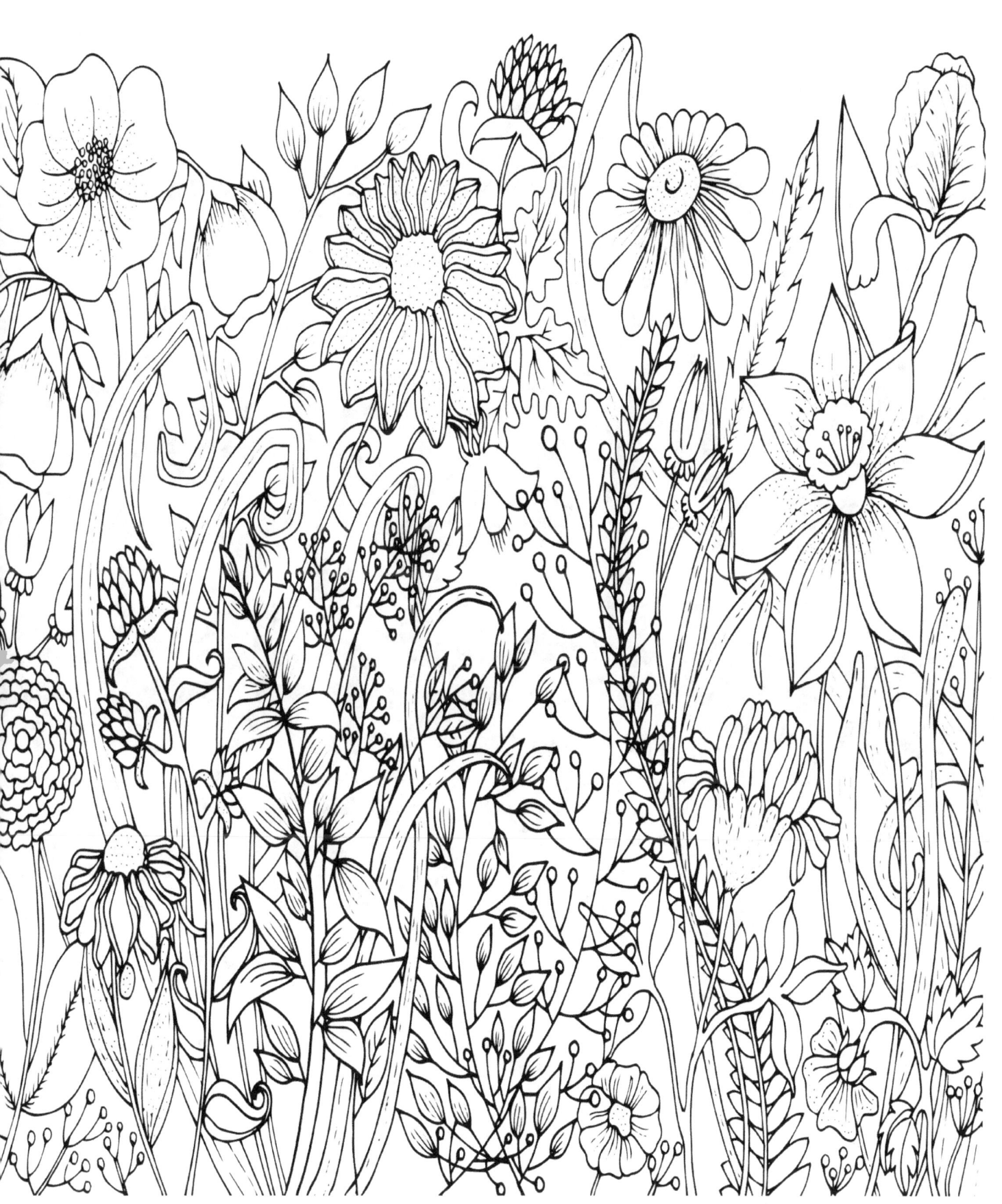

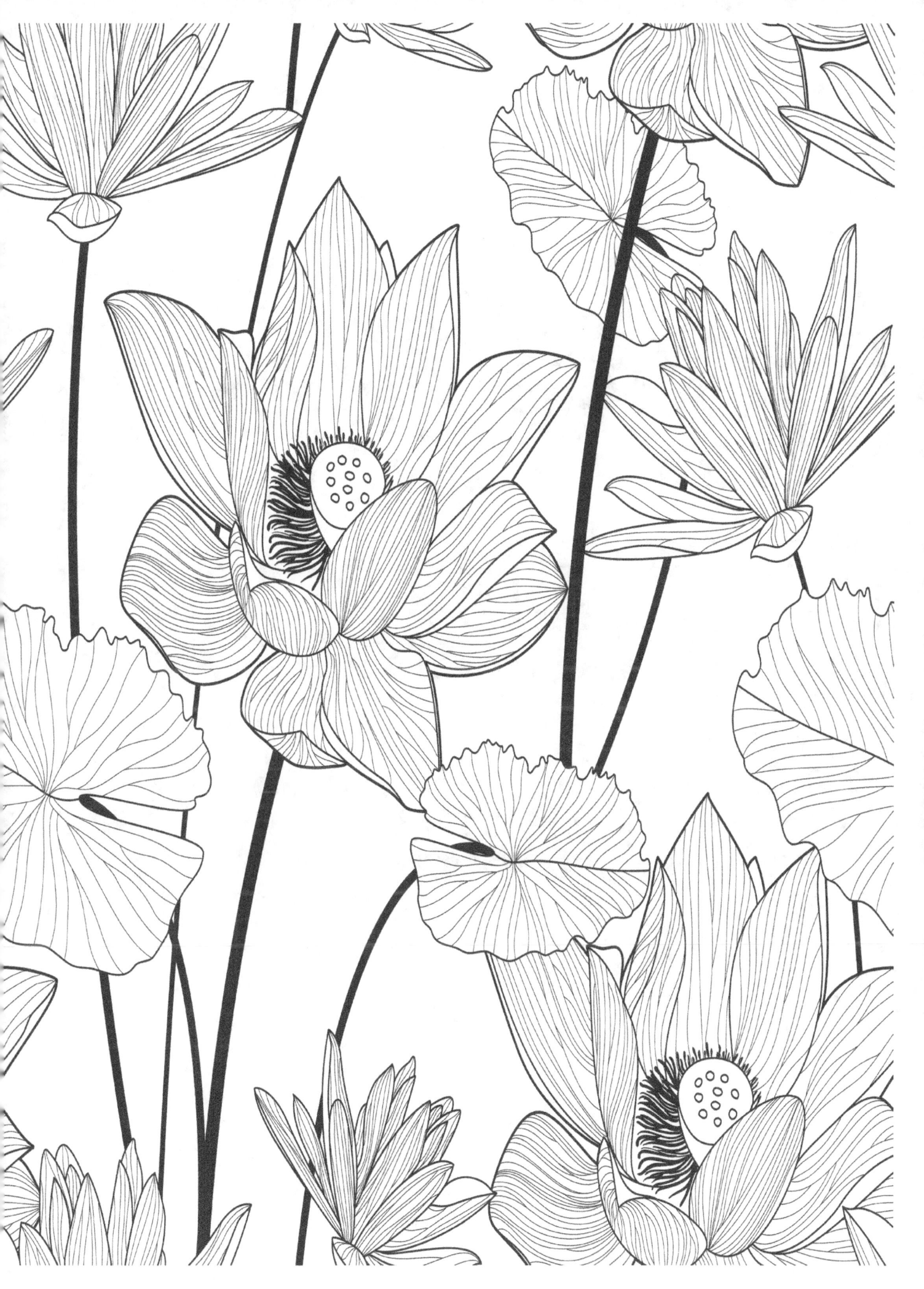

www.ingramcontent.com/pod-product-compliance
Lightning Source LLC
Chambersburg PA
CBHW081301180526
45170CB00007B/2513